# SLOW COOKER COOKBOOK FOR TWO

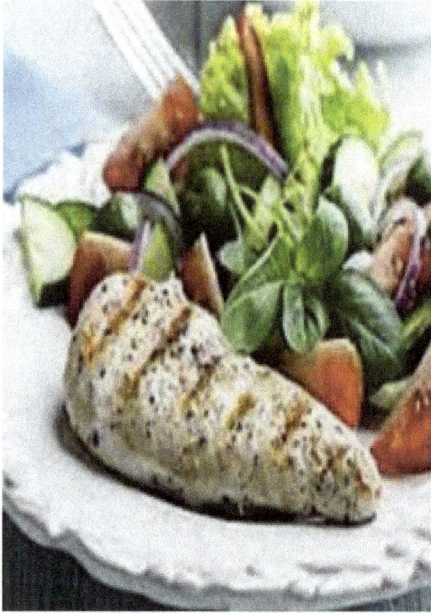
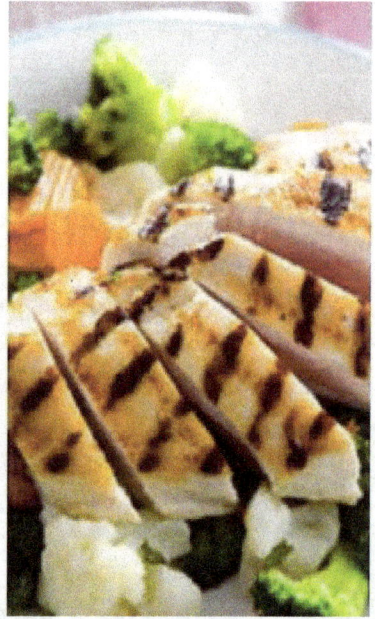
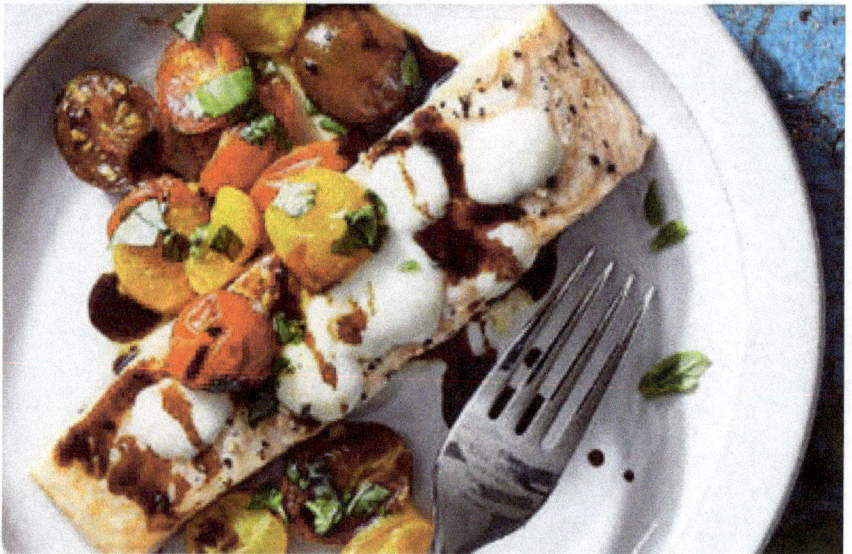

# Table of Contents

# INTRODUCTION

A slow cooker can prove to be useful with a tasty feast sitting tight for you and your family toward the day's end.

Slow Cooker Tips and Safety

In the event that you are reluctant to have your slow cooker on and cooking while you are away for the duration of the day, consider cooking food sources during substitute hours that you are home, even while you rest. Cool down the food varieties when they are done cooking, putting away it in the fridge before reheating it in the oven or oven for a feast later.

Here are some fundamental tips and security rules to follow when using a slow cooker:

For simple cleanup and care of your slow cooker, rub within the stoneware with oil or splash it with nonstick cooking shower prior to using it. Slow cooker liners additionally ease cleanup.

Continuously defrost frozen meat and poultry in the fridge prior to cooking it in the slow cooker. To guarantee total cooking, don't place frozen meat in your slow cooker.

Fill the slow cooker no not exactly half full and close to 66% full. Cooking nearly nothing or an excessive amount of food in the slow cooker can influence cooking time, quality and the security.

Since vegetables cook slower than meat and poultry, place the vegetables in the slow cooker first. Spot the meat on top of the vegetables and top with fluid, like stock, water or a sauce.

Add the fluid, like stock, water or grill sauce, recommended in the formula. Since fluids don't reduce away in a slow cooker, much of the time, you can lessen fluids by 33% to one-half while changing over a non-slow cooker formula for slow cooker use.

In the event that conceivable, set your slow cooker on high for the primary hour, and afterward turn the heat setting too low to get done with cooking.

# Slow cooker meals

## 20+ recipes

# 1.    Braised pork with plums

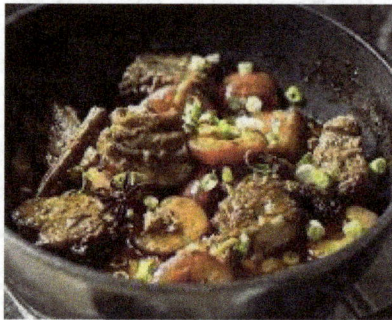

Prep: 25 mins | Cook: 2 hrs. | Plus marinating | Serves 8

## Ingredients

- about 1.6kg/3lb 8oz pork shoulder
- 5 tbsp. rice wine
- 5 tbsp. light soy sauce for flavor, 1 tbsp. dull for shading
- liberal thumb-size piece new root ginger
- 5 garlic cloves
- 1 red stew , deseeded and finely chopped
- 2 tbsp. vegetable oil
- pack spring onions , finely cut
- 2 star anise
- 1 ½ tsp. five-flavor powder

- 1 cinnamon stick
- 2 tbsp. sugar , any sort
- 1 tbsp. tomato purée
- 500ml chicken stock
- 6 ready plums , split and stoned

## Strategy

1. Cut the pork into huge pieces about the length of your thumb and twice as wide. Put into a bowl or food pack, and add the wine, soy sauces, a large portion of the ginger, a large portion of the garlic and a large portion of the bean stew. Marinate for in any event 1 hr. or up to 24 hrs.
2. Heat oven to 160C/140C fan/gas 3, at that point heat the oil in a large goulash. Tip down the middle the spring onions, staying ginger and garlic, the star anise, five-zest powder and cinnamon. Fry tenderly until fragrant and delicate. Mix in the sugar, turn up the heat, at that point lift the pork from the marinade and turn in the oniony blend for around 3 mins until the meat is simply fixed yet not browned. Tip in the marinade, tomato purée and stock, give it a mix, cover, at that point braise in the oven for 2 hrs.
3. After the main hr. is up, add the plums to the container. Take the cover off and carry on the cooking, revealed. The meat ought to be totally delicate, becoming brilliant brown where it breaks the outside of the sauce. Spoon off any overabundance fat from the surface, at that point scoop the meat and plums cautiously from the dish with an opened spoon.

Turn up the heat and heat up the sauce for 5-10 mins until decreased and somewhat sweet. Return everything to the dish, delicately warm through; at that point disperse the remainder of the spring onions over the top to serve.

4. Formula TIPS
5. In the event that YOU WANT TO USE A SLOW COOKER...
6. Adjust this formula by setting up the pork as indicated by stage 1. At that point cook the spring onions, staying ginger, garlic, stew, cinnamon, star anise, five-zest, and sugar and 2 tbsp. tomato purée. Fry until delicate at that point add the pork, singing until fixed. Put everything into the slow cooker with the marinade and stock, cover and cook for 8-9 hours on Low. Skim off surface fat partially through. Mix in the plums an hour prior as far as possible. Scoop out the plums and meat at that point makes the sauce and serves as per stage 3.

# 2.   Cottage pie

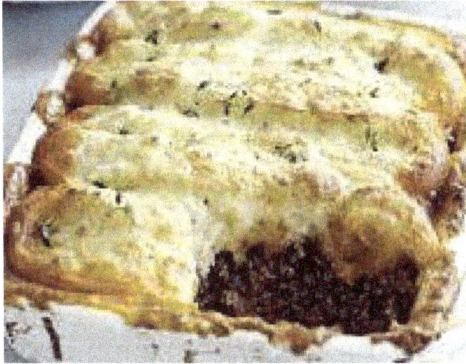

Prep: 35 mins | Cook: 1 hr. and 50 mins | Serves 10

## *Ingredients*

- 3 tbsp. olive oil
- 1 ¼kg hamburger mince
- 2 onions, finely chopped
- 3 carrots, chopped
- 3 celery sticks, chopped
- 2 garlic cloves, finely chopped
- 3 tbsp. plain flour
- 1 tbsp. tomato purée
- large glass red wine (discretionary)
- 850ml hamburger stock
- 4 tbsp. Worcestershire sauce
- not many thyme twigs
- 2 narrows leaves
- For the pound
- 1.8kg potatoes, chopped
- 225ml milk
- 25g margarine
- 200g solid cheddar, ground
- newly ground nutmeg

### Technique

1. Heat 1 tbsp. olive oil in a large pan and fry 1¼ kg hamburger mince until browned – you may have to do this in clusters. Put away as it browns.
2. Put the other 2 tbsp. olive oil into the skillet, add 2 finely chopped onions, 3 chopped carrots and 3 chopped celery sticks and cook on a delicate heat until delicate, around 20 mins.
3. Add 2 finely chopped garlic cloves, 3 tbsp. plain flour and 1 tbsp. tomato purée, increment the heat and cook for a couple of mins, at that point return the meat to the container.
4. Pour over a large glass of red wine, if using, and bubble to diminish it marginally prior to adding the 850ml meat stock, 4 tbsp. Worcestershire sauce, a couple of thyme twigs and 2 cove leaves.
5. Bring to a stew and cook, uncovered, for 45 mins. At this point the sauce ought to be thick and covering the meat. Check after around 30 mins – if a ton of fluid remaining parts, increment the heat marginally to lessen the sauce a bit. Season well, at that point disposes of the cove leaves and thyme stalks.
6. In the interim, make the crush. In a large pan, cover the 1.8kg potatoes which you've stripped and chopped, in salted virus water, bring to the bubble and stew until delicate.
7. Channel well, at that point permits to steam-dry for a couple of mins. Squash well with the 225ml milk, 25g margarine, and 3/4 of the 200g solid cheddar, at that point season with

newly ground nutmeg and some salt and pepper.

8. Spoon the meat into 2 ovenproof dishes. Line or spoon on the squash to cover. Sprinkle on the excess cheddar.

9. In the case of consuming straight, heat oven to 220C/200C fan/gas 7 and cook for 25-30 mins or until the garnish is brilliant.

10. On the off chance that you need to utilize a slow cooker, brown your mince in clumps at that point tip into your slow cooker and mix in the vegetables, flour, purée, wine, stock, Worcestershire sauce and spices with some flavoring. Cover and cook on High for 4-5 hours. Make the crush following the past advances, and afterward oven cook similarly to wrap up.


11. Formula TIPS

12. OUR TOP TIPS

13. To get truly smooth, rich squash, utilize a potato ricer or strainer. To stop the pound sinking into the filling, permit the meat to cool prior to garnish with the squashed potato. Freeze in individual ovenproof dishes for a simple supper for one. For a truly fresh, brilliant garnish, streak under the barbecue for a couple of mins prior to serving.

14. Secure FREEZING

15. Ensure the pie is totally cool, at that point cover it well with stick film and freeze. Continuously freeze the pie on the day that you make it. Thaw out in the ice chest short-

term; at that point cook according to the formula. Then again, to cook from frozen, heat oven to 180C/160C fan/gas 4, cover with foil and cook for 1½ hrs. Increment oven to 220C/200C fan/gas 7, uncover and cook for 20 mins more, until brilliant and gurgling.

# 3. Golden veggie shepherd's pie

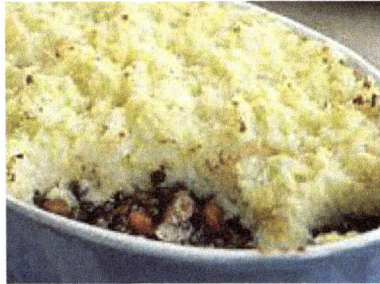

Preparation and cooking time | Prep: 30 mins |
Cook: 1 hr. and 45 mins | Serves 10

## *Ingredients*
For the lentil sauce
50g margarine
2 onions, chopped
4 carrots, diced
1 head of celery, chopped
4 garlic cloves, finely chopped
200g pack chestnut mushrooms, cut
2 cove leaves
1 tbsp. dried thyme
500g pack dried green lentils (we utilized Merchant Gourmet Pay lentils)
100ml red wine (discretionary)
1.7L vegetable stock
3 tbsp. tomato purée
For the garnish
2kg floury potato, like King Edwards
85g spread
100ml milk
50g cheddar, ground

## Technique

1. To make the sauce, heat 50g spread in a container, at that point tenderly fry 2 chopped onions, 4 diced carrots, 1 chopped head of celery and 4 finely chopped garlic cloves for 15 mins until delicate and brilliant.
2. Turn up the heat, add 200g cut chestnut mushrooms, and at that point cook for 4 mins more.
3. Mix in 2 straight leaves and 1 tbsp. dried thyme; at that point add 500g green lentils. Pour over 100ml red wine and 1.7l vegetable stock – it's significant that you don't prepare with salt at this stage.
4. Stew for 40-50 mins until the lentils are extremely delicate.
5. Season to taste, take off heat, and at that point mix in 3 tbsp. tomato purée.
6. While the lentils are cooking, tip 2kg floury potatoes into a dish of water, at that point bubble for around 15 mins until delicate. Channel well, crush with 85g spread and 100ml milk, at that point season with salt and pepper.
7. To collect the pies, split the lentil combination between every one of the dishes that you are using, at that point top with pound.
8. Dissipate over 50g ground cheddar and freeze for as long as two months or assuming eating that day, heat oven to 190C/fan 170C/gas 5, prepare for 30 mins until the fixing is brilliant.
9. Formula TIPS
10. COOKING INSTRUCTIONS

11. For best outcomes, thaw out the readied pies altogether prior to cooking as expressed. The pies can likewise be cooked from frozen if shy of time – first heat oven to 160C/fan 140C/gas 3, at that point cover the pie with thwart and prepare for 1 hr-1 hr. 20 mins (30 mins for singular pies) until totally delicate when nudged with a blade. Increment the heat to 200C/fan 180C/gas 6, reveal, and at that point keep on cooking for 20 mins until brilliant on top and steaming hot.
12. LENTILS
13. You could likewise utilize three jars of washed and depleted green lentils for this – basically make the stock, at that point stew them for only 10 minutes.
14. Instructions to FREEZE
15. On the off chance that you have bunches of pie dishes, you can make the pies in an assortment of sizes to suit various events, at that point freeze them. I like to make two large pies to serve up to four, in addition to two individual pies – ideal for an independent dinner or a heavenly dinner for the sitter. In the event that you don't have heaps of dishes, you can freeze the sauce, squash and cheddar in isolated cooler sacks, at that point thaw out and gather when required.
16. In the event that YOU WANT TO USE A SLOW COOKER...
17. Fry off your onions, celery, carrots and garlic for 15 mins in a skillet. Tip into your slow cooker with the mushrooms, spices and lentils. Pour over the stock and wine, cover and cook

on High for 5-6 hours. In the mean time make the squashed potato as per stage 6. Mood killer the slow cooker, season and mix in the tomato purée. Proceed from stage 7, splitting the lentils between dishes, top with the pound and cheddar and cook for 30 mins until quite hot.

# 4.  Rich paprika seafood bowl

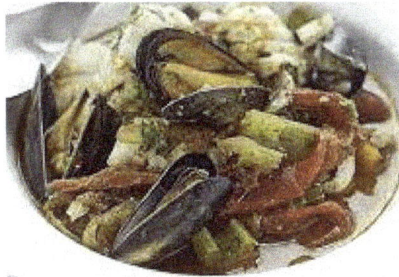

Prep: 10 mins | Cook: 20 mins | Serves 4

## Ingredients

- 1 tbsp. olive oil
- 2 onions , divided and meagerly cut
- 2 celery stems, finely chopped
- large bundle level leaf parsley , leaves and stalks isolated
- 2-3 tsp. paprika
- 200g broiled red pepper , depleted weight, thickly cut
- 400g can chopped tomato with garlic
- 400g white fish filet, cut into exceptionally large lumps
- barely any new mussels (discretionary)

## Technique

1. Heat the oil in a container, at that point add the onions, celery and somewhat salt. Cover, at that point delicately fry until delicate, around 10 mins. Put the parsley stalks, a large portion of the leaves, oil and preparing into a food processor and whizz to a paste. Add this and the paprika to the relaxed onions, broiling for a couple of mins. Tip in the peppers and tomatoes with a sprinkle of water; at that point stew for 10 mins until the sauce has decreased.
2. Lay the fish and mussels on top of the sauce, put a cover on, and at that point stew for 5 mins until the fish is simply chipping and the mussels have opened – dispose of any that stay shut. Tenderly mix the fish into the sauce, season, at that point serve in bowls.
3. Formula TIPS
4. On the off chance that YOU WANT TO USE A SLOW COOKER...
5. Leave this stew to implant for more. Whizz the parsley stalks, a large portion of the leaves, oil and preparing in a food processor. Add this to the onions, celery, paprika, peppers and tomatoes in the slow cooker pot. Cook on Low for 8-10 hours. Settle the mussels in the sauce and dissipate the fish on top. Re-cover and cook on High for 30 mins 60 minutes. Dispose of any unopened mussels, mix the fish into the sauce at that point serve.
6. Works out positively For
7. Peach and almond crunch

# 5.   Creamy veggie korma

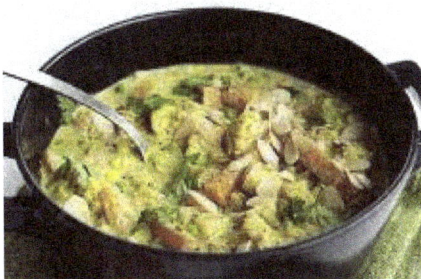

Prep: 15 mins | Cook: 30 mins | Serves 4

## Ingredients

- 1 tbsp. vegetable oil
- 1 onion, finely chopped
- 3 cardamom cases, slammed
- 2 tsp. each ground cumin and coriander
- ½ tsp. ground turmeric
- 1 green bean stew, deseeded (whenever wanted) and finely chopped
- 1 garlic clove, squashed
- thumb-size piece ginger, finely chopped
- 800g blended vegetable, like carrots, cauliflower, potato and corvette, chopped
- 300-500ml hot vegetable stock
- 200g frozen peas
- 200ml yogurt
- 2 tbsp. ground almonds (discretionary)
- Make it non-veggie
- ½ little crude chicken bosom per divide
- To serve
- toasted chipped almonds, chopped coriander, basmati rice or naan bread

### Strategy

1. Heat the oil in a large dish. Cook onion with the dry flavors over a low heat for 5-6 mins until the onion is light brilliant. Add the bean stew, garlic and ginger and cook for 1 min, at that point toss in the blended vegetables and cook for a further 5 mins.

2. Gap the blend fittingly between two dishes if serving veggie lovers and meat eaters. Slash the chicken into little pieces and mix into one dish. Add the stock, splitting between the dish properly, and stew for 10 mins (if just cooking the veggie rendition in one skillet, utilize 300ml stock; if splitting between two container, add 250ml to each). Gap the peas, if fundamental, and add, cooking for 3 mins more until the veg are delicate and the chicken is cooked through.

3. Eliminate from the heat and mix through the yogurt and ground almonds, if using. Serve sprinkled with the toasted almonds and coriander, with basmati rice or naan bread as an afterthought.

4. Formula TIPS

5. On the off chance that YOU WANT TO USE A SLOW COOKER...

6. On the off chance that you need to make the vegan rendition of this curry in a slow cooker, right off the bat cook off the onions with the dry flavors in a griddle for 5-6 mins. Add the bean stew, garlic and ginger and cook for 1 moment, at that point tip into your slow cooker. Toss in the vegetables and 400ml stock, cover and cook on Low for 4 hours until

the potatoes are delicate. Mix in the peas, yogurt and ground almonds with preparing, represent 5 minutes at that point fill in as above.

7. Works out in a good way For
8. One skillet fiery rice

# 6.    Slow cooker lamb kolifto

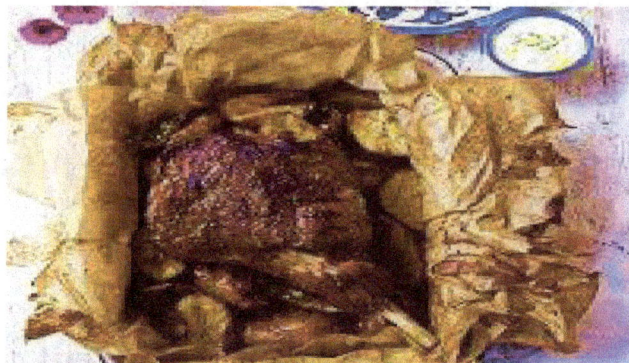

5 Hours + Marinating Serves 4

## Ingredients

- Lemon 1 enormous, squeezed
- Extra-virgin olive oil 100ml
- Dry white wine 175ml
- Dark peppercorns squashed to make ½ tsp.
- Garlic 4 cloves, stripped and left entirety
- Dried oregano 2 tsp.
- Ground cumin 1 tsp.
- Sheep shanks 4
- Ocean salt drops 1 tsp.
- Ready tomato 1 enormous, cut into quarters
- Cinnamon stick 1
- Waxy potatoes 750g, stripped and cut into reduced down 3D squares
- Level leaf parsley a modest bunch, generally chopped

## Directions:

1. Put the lemon juice, 2 tbsp. oil, wine, pepper, garlic, oregano and cumin into a blender and whizz. Put the shanks into a bowl, pour over the marinade and back rub well to cover. Cover and chill for at any rate 1 hour yet ideally overnight.
2. Heat the slow cooker to high or low, contingent upon wanted cooking time.
3. Put the meat, marinade, salt, tomato and cinnamon stick into the slow cooker. Cover with the top and cook for 3-4 hours on high, or 6-8 hours on low until totally delicate.
4. At the point when the sheep is cooked through and totally delicate, earthy colored the potatoes in 3 tbsp. of olive oil in a griddle over a medium-high heat until they start to shading and relax.
5. Eliminate the sheep from the slow cooker, put on a plate and cover firmly with foil.
6. Add the seared potatoes to the slow cooker and blend well. Cover and keep cooking for an additional 45 minutes-1 hour or until the potatoes are cooked and delicate. Add the sheep back to the slow cooker to heat through again. Check the flavoring, adding more if vital.
7. Present with hard bread and a green serving of mixed greens.

# 7. Slow-cooked duck legs in Port with celeriac gratin

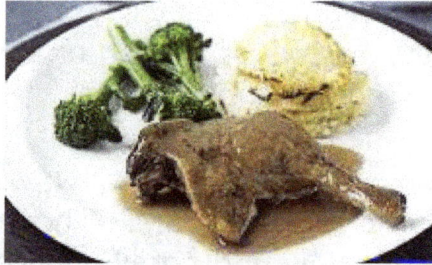

Cook: 2 hrs. and 30 mins | Prep 15 mins + infusing |
Serves 2

## *Ingredients*

- 2 duck legs
- 2 carrots , generally chopped
- 1 little onion , generally chopped
- 1 tbsp. plain flour
- 1 cove leaf
- 1 star anise
- 2 cloves
- 2 strips orange skin (with a potato peeler)
- 150ml port
- 500ml chicken stock
- For the gratin
- 100ml milk
- 100ml twofold cream
- 1 garlic clove , crushed.
- 1 rosemary branch
- 25g margarine , in addition to extra for lubing
- ¼ little celeriac (about 100g), quartered and meagerly cut
- 1 little potato , meagerly cut

- ground parmesan , for sprinkling
- occasional vegetables , to serve

## *Technique*

1. Heat oven to 160C/140C fan/gas 3. Put the duck legs in a flameproof goulash set over a medium heat. Brown all finished, at that point eliminate from the goulash and put away. Pour off everything except 1 tbsp. of the fat, leave more fat in the skillet on the off chance that you are multiplying or significantly increasing (save the depleted fat for your Christmas roasties). Add the carrots and onion to the goulash and cook for 5-10 mins or until beginning to caramelize. Mix in the flour and cook for 1 min more. Return the duck alongside the excess ingredients. Bring to a stew, at that point cover with a top and put in the oven for 2 hrs.

2. In the interim, set up the gratin. Put the milk, cream, garlic and rosemary in a dish set over a low heat. Bring to a delicate stew for 5 mins, at that point eliminate from the heat and leave to implant for 30 mins. Oil 2 ramekins (about 8cm breadth, 5cm profound). Mastermind the celeriac and potato cuts in the ramekins, preparing the layers as you go. Eliminate the garlic and rosemary from the milk, pour over the veg, at that point dab with spread. Cover firmly with thwart and prepare with the duck for 1½ hrs.

3. When cooked, eliminate the duck and gratins from the oven. To freeze the duck, cool, at that point pack into a cooler holder, pushing the

duck under the sauce. On the off chance that it doesn't cover it, lay stick film on top. Use inside 2 months. Defrost in the ice chest, at that point reheat in the meal and complete from Step 4. Increment oven to 220C/200C fan/gas 7. Put a hefty can on top of each foil-wrapped gratin and represent 15-20 mins, or chill like this until required. When squeezed, turn the gratins out onto a heating plate, sprinkle with a little Parmesan and prepare for 20 mins until brilliant.

4. In the interim, eliminate the duck legs from the goulash, strain the cooking fluid into a perfect container and bring to a fast bubble. Diminish the sauce significantly until thickened and polished. Add the duck legs and heat through. Put a duck leg on each plate with a little sauce spooned over the top. Present with the gratins and occasional veg.

# 8. Slow-cooked Greek Easter lamb with lemons, olives & bay

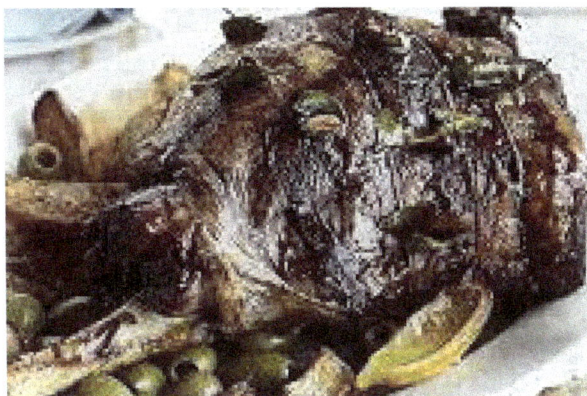

Prep: 20 mins | Cook: 4 hrs. and 30 mins | plus resting | Serves 6

## Ingredients

- 1 garlic bulb , isolated into cloves, half stripped and cut, half unpeeled
- 8-10 new inlet leaves
- 3 lemons , cut into quarters lengthways
- 2 ½kg leg of sheep
- 50ml Greek additional virgin olive oil , in addition to 4 tbsp. for the potatoes
- 1 tsp. ground cinnamon
- 1kg Cypriot potatoes , stripped and quartered lengthways (in the event that you can't track down these, any large, waxy assortment is fine – attempt Desiree)
- 140g Greek Kalkidis olives (or other large hollowed green olives)
- 125ml red or dry white wine

## Technique

1. Heat oven to 220C/200C fan/gas 7. Mastermind the unpeeled garlic cloves, 3 straight leaves and the lemon quarters in a large broiling dish and cover with 200ml virus water. Sit the sheep on top, shower with the olive oil and focus on everything over.
2. Using a little sharp blade, cut little cuts in the sheep skin, at that point fold the excess stripped and cut garlic and inlet leaves into these cuts.
3. Season the sheep well and sprinkle over the cinnamon. Cover firmly with foil and spot in the oven. Promptly diminish the oven temperature to 150C/130C fan/gas 2. Leave to cook for 4 hrs., skimming the fat from the juices and eliminating the foil for the last 30 mins of cooking.
4. After 1 hr., put the potato wedges in a large broiling tin, coat those in 4 tbsp. olive oil and season well. Broil in the oven with the sheep for 11/2-2 hrs.
5. Move the cooked sheep to a large part of foil wrap firmly and leave to rest for 20-30 mins. Check the potatoes are cooked (on the off chance that you need to, turn the oven up to 220C/200C fan/gas 7 to get done with cooking). Add the olives and wine to the container juices, stew them and keep warm until prepared to cut. Serve the sheep thickly cut with the olives, potatoes and Tahini and lemon sauce (see 'works out in a good way for'), with the meat juices pored over without a second to spare.

6. Formula TIPS
7. ADD A GARLIC HIT
8. For an additional hit of garlic, tenderly press the broiled (unpeeled) garlic cloves from the lower part of the dish with the rear of a spoon while the sheep rests. Blend the garlic into the dish juices prior to pouring over the meat.
9. Works out positively For
10. Tahini and lemon sauce
11. Spinach rice
12. Goliath spread bean stew

# 9.  Slow-cooked celeriac with pork & orange

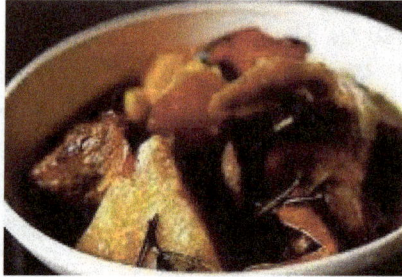

Total time3 hrs. | Ready in 2½-3 hrs. including 2 hours in the oven | More effort | Serves 2

## *Ingredients*
- 3 leeks , managed and washed
- 2 carrots , stripped
- 3 tbsp. olive oil
- 900g boneless pork , cut into large stewing pieces (shoulder is an ideal sliced to utilize)
- 2 little or 1 large celeriac (about 1kg/2lb 4oz), stripped and diced into large pieces
- 2 garlic cloves , chopped
- 200ml dry white wine
- 200ml chicken stock
- squeeze and zing of 1 orange (eliminate the orange zing with a potato peeler)
- 2 tsp. soy sauce
- large twig of rosemary
- dried up bread , to serve

## Strategy

1. Preheat the oven to fan 120C/regular 140C/gas 1. Cut every leek into around five pieces, hack the carrots into pieces similar size as the leeks. Heat a large, lidded, flameproof meal dish on the hob until it's hot. Add 2 tbsp. of the olive oil at that point cautiously tip the pork into the meal and leave it several minutes to brown. Mix once, at that point leaves for several minutes. Using an opened spoon, move the meat to a plate. Pour the remainder of the oil into the dish, tip in the leeks, carrots and celeriac and fry for 3-4 minutes, mixing, until they begin to brown. Add the garlic and fry briefly more.

2. Mix the pork and any juices into the vegetables, at that point pour in the wine, stock, squeezed orange and soy sauce. Toss in the rosemary and orange zing, season with salt and pepper, give it a mix, and at that point carry everything to the bubble.

3. Cover the dish, move it to the oven and cook for 2 hours, mixing following 60 minutes. Cook until the pork is delicate and the leeks self-destruct when pushed with a spoon. (It would now be able to be left to cool and afterward frozen for as long as multi month.) Leave to represent at any rate 10 minutes, at that point spoon into bowls. Present with hard bread to absorb each one of those juices.

# 10. Slow cooker chickpea Dahl

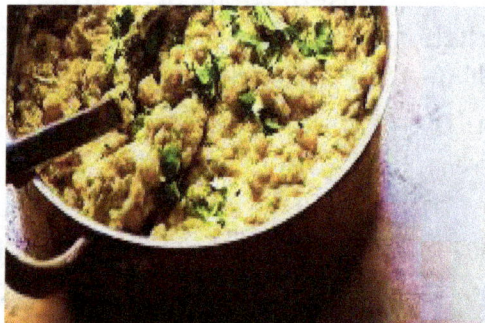

2 Hours 30 Minutes + Proving Serves 8

## *Ingredients*

- sunflower oil
- onions 2 large, slashed
- ginger 50g, peeled and grated
- Ground cumin 1 tbsp.
- Ground coriander 1 tbsp.
- nigella seeds 1 tbsp., plus more for the naans
- Medium curry powder 1 tbsp.
- Turmeric 1 tsp.
- red split lentils 300g
- chana Dahl (dried split chickpeas) 500g
- coconut milk 2 x 400g tins
- NAANS
- fast-action dried yeast 7g
- natural yogurt 100g
- strong white bread flour 500g, plus more for dusting
- Fine salt 1½ tsp.

- clarified butter or ghee

## DIRECTIONS:

1. To make the naans, blend the yeast and yogurt in with 250ml warm water. Put the flour and salt in a bowl and bit by bit mix in the yeast blend until it meets up as a batter. Tip out onto the work surface and massage for 10 minutes, or 5 minutes in a blender with the mixture snare, until smooth. Put into a perfect bowl, cover with oiled Clingfilm and leave for 2 hours, or until multiplied in size.

2. Heat 1 tbsp. oil in a huge skillet, and fry the onion and ginger until truly delicate. Mix in the flavors, cook for brief at that point add the lentils and chana Dahl. Add the coconut milk, 800ml water and some flavoring. Bring to a stew, go down to a low heat and cook for 1½ hours, covered, blending delicately from time to time, adding more water if necessary. To freeze, cool the Dahl totally, tip into compartments and put in the cooler.

3. At the point when the mixture is prepared, manipulate it momentarily on a softly floured work surface. Cut into 8 pieces and carry everyone out to an oval until they done spring back. Lay onto oiled preparing sheets, cover with oiled Clingfilm and leave for 30 minutes until puffy.

4. Heat the oven to 240C/fan 220C/gas 9. Heat another preparing sheet in the oven. Move the naans, two all at once, onto the hot preparing sheet. Cook for 5-10 minutes until the batter begins to bubble and the base looks brilliant.

Press them tenderly back down on the off chance that they've domed to an extreme. Cool under a perfect tea towel, at that point exclusively envelop by foil and freeze.

5.  To reheat, thaw out the Dahl in the cooler short-term, and leave the naans on the work surface to come to room temperature. Heat the oven to 220C/fan 200C/gas 7. Put the Dahl into a dish with a sprinkle of water, bring to a stew and cook until steaming hot. Put the naans on a heating sheet, sprinkle with a little water and reheat in the oven for 5 minutes or until warmed through. Brush the naans with explained margarine or ghee, and disperse over some nigella seeds to serve.

6.  Put all the Dahl ingredients and 800ml water in a slow cooker. Cook on high for 3 1/2 – 4 hours until the lentils are delicate.

# 11. Caramelised squash & spinach lasagna

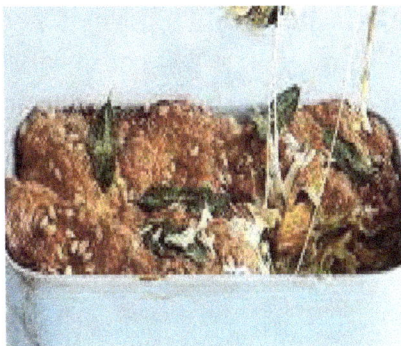

Prep: 25 mins | Cook: 1 hr. and 40 mins | plus cooling | Serves 6

## Ingredients

- 1 medium butternut squash, stripped, seeds eliminated and cut into 2cm 3D squares (1.2kg arranged weight)
- 3 garlic cloves, unpeeled
- modest bunch of sage leaves
- 1 tbsp. olive oil, in addition to a little extra
- 600g new spinach
- 12-15 lasagne sheets
- 125g ball mozzarella, torn or cut into little pieces
- 40g pine nuts
- For the white sauce
- 70g margarine
- 70g flour
- 800ml milk
- 250g mascarpone

- 50g parmesan (or veggie lover elective), ground
- grinding of nutmeg

### *Strategy*

1. Heat the oven to 200C/180C fan/gas 6. Tip the squash and garlic into a large cooking tin or dish (you can utilize a similar one to amass the lasagne to save money on cleaning up – our own was 35 x 40cm and 5cm profound). Tear more than 4-5 sage leaves, shower with the oil and season well, and at that point throw to cover. Cook for 40-50 mins, moving the squash around more than once, until delicate and caramelized. Crush the garlic from the skins and pound with the squash, leaving a couple of stout pieces for surface.

2. In the mean time, make the white sauce. Soften the spread in a large pot, and mix in the flour to make a sandy paste. Sprinkle a little milk into the dish, blending constantly to forestall bumps. Continue to add more milk, a little at a time, until the paste diminishes to a smooth, rich sauce and the milk has all been utilized. Stew for 1 min more. Mix in the mascarpone and a large portion of the parmesan. Season well and mesh in a liberal measure of nutmeg.

3. Tip the spinach into a colander and pour over a kettleful of bubbling water to shrink (do this in clumps). When sufficiently cool to deal with, crush the spinach over the colander to eliminate the water, at that point season and generally cleave.

4. Eliminate half of the squashed garlicky squash from the cooking tin and put away on a plate. Spread the excess squash out over the base of the tin or dish you mean to serve the lasagne in. Spoon over about a fourth of the sauce, at that point top with a solitary layer of lasagne sheets, snapping them to fill any holes. Make an even layer of spinach on top of the pasta, and top with another quarter of the sauce, more pasta, squash, sauce, pasta lastly the excess white sauce.
5. Disperse over the leftover parmesan, the mozzarella and pine nuts. On the off chance that the oven is off, heat to 200C/180C fan/gas 6 and cook the lasagne for 30 mins. Rub some additional oil more than 5 or 6 sage leaves, place them on top of the lasagne and get back to the oven for another 15-20 mins until brilliant and percolating. Leave to cool for 5 mins prior to serving.
6. Works out in a good way For
7. Slow-cooked stout meat lasagne
8. Green plate of mixed greens with olive dressing
9. Green plate of mixed greens with buttermilk dressing.

# 12. Lamb bhuna

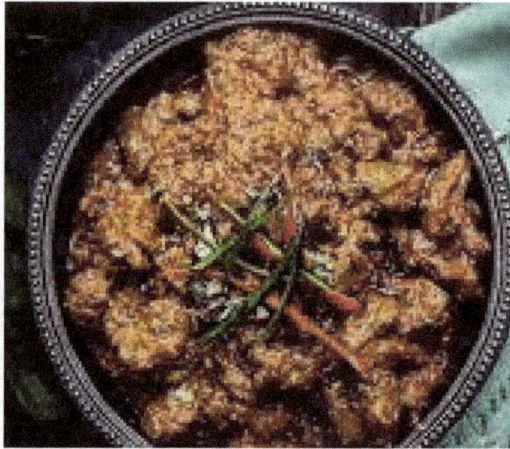

Prep: 30 mins | Cook: 1 hr. and 40 min| plus at least 1 hr. marinating | More effort | Serves 4

## *Ingredients*

- 600g sheep neck filet or shoulder, cut into large lumps
- For the marinade
- 6 garlic cloves, finely ground
- thumb-sized piece of ginger, stripped and finely ground
- 2 tbsp. malt vinegar
- ½ tsp. ground cinnamon
- 1 tbsp. sunflower oil
- For the sauce
- 3 tbsp. sunflower oil, in addition to some extra if necessary
- 2 onions, finely chopped
- 10 curry leaves
- 2 dried chilies, or ½ tsp. stew drops
- 1 tsp. cumin seeds
- 1 tsp. mustard seeds

- 1 tsp. ground coriander
- ½ tsp. fenugreek seeds or ground fenugreek
- 1 tbsp. tomato purée
- 400g can chopped tomatoes
- 1 tsp. gram masala

## Strategy

1. To make the marinade, consolidate the ingredients with a large touch of salt in a large bowl. Throw in the sheep, cover and marinate for 1 hr. at room temperature, or chill for the time being.
2. For the sauce, heat the oil in a flameproof meal and fry the onions for 10 mins, blending until delicate and brilliant. Shower in more oil if the dish gets dry. Add the curry leaves and chilies and fry for a couple of moments, at that point add the flavors and cook for 5 mins more until the onions begin to caramelize.
3. Tip in the sheep alongside the marinade and turn the heat to high. Cook, mixing, for 5 mins until the sheep browns. Add the tomato purée and cook for 1 min, at that point mix in the tomatoes and 100ml water. Bring to a stew, decrease the heat, cover and cook, mixing every so often, for 1 hr. 20 mins until the sheep is delicate.
4. Reveal and cook for 8-10 mins more until the sauce has decreased and thickened. Eliminate from the heat, mix in the garam masalaa and season. Will keep chilled for as long as three days or frozen for a very long time.
5. Works out in a good way For
6. Carrot pakoras

7. Paneer and chickpea fry
8. Fast and puffy flatbreads

# 13. Herb-scented slow-roasted rib of beef

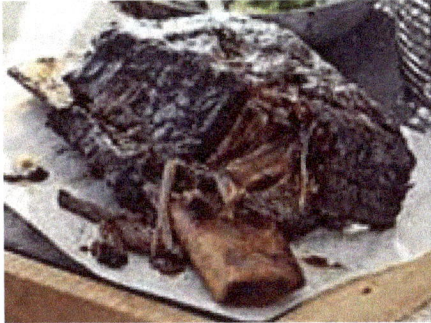

Prep: 30 mins | Cook: 5 hrs. | Plus at least 3 hrs. to bring to room temperature and resting | More effort | Serves 10

## *Ingredients*

- 3-bone rib of hamburger joint (around 3-3.5kg)
- 4 garlic cloves , left entire however slammed once
- 4 rosemary twigs
- ½ pack thyme
- small bunch inlet leaves
- 4 allspice berries
- 4 cloves
- 1 tsp. dark peppercorns
- 200ml red wine
- 1 tbsp. plain flour
- For the coating
- 2 tbsp. Bovril
- 2 tbsp. Dijon mustard
- 1 tbsp. dark remedy

### Technique

1. Remove the hamburger from the cooler and surrender it to come to temperature short-term or for at any rate three hours. Tip the garlic and every one of the spices and flavors into a large simmering tin and, using a blow light or under a hot flame broil, burn the spices until they begin to seethe (in the event that using a barbecue to do this, don't leave it unattended), leave to cool marginally.

2. Heat oven to 100C/80C fan/gas ¼. Rub a tbsp. of salt over the meat; at that point sit the joint on top of the spices. Pour over the wine; at that point firmly tent the tin two or three sheets of extra-wide foil. Cook in the oven for 1 hr., at that point lessen the temperature to 70C/50C fan (on the off chance that you have a gas oven, don't change the temperature), and slow dish for 3 hrs. more.

3. Eliminate the foil, at that point embed a computerized test into the center of the joint – when the temperature stretches around 60C, it's prepared. In the event that the meat isn't up to temperature, increment oven to 150C/130C fan/gas 2, and meal with the foil off, checking the temperature each 15 mins. While the hamburger is cooking, make the coating by whisking every one of the ingredients together.

4. At the point when the hamburger is cooked, eliminate from the oven and increment the temperature to 230C/210C fan/gas 8. Return the hamburger to the oven for 5 mins to fresh and rankle the fat, at that point liberally brush

the coating everywhere on the joint and get back to the oven for 5 mins until tacky and slightly singed – watch out for it, as it will consume effectively at this stage. Lift the meat onto a slashing load up and leave to rest for 20 mins.

5. To make a herby sauce, put the broiling tin over a low heat and mix in the flour to make a gloopy paste. Include any excess coating, at that point cautiously pour in 500ml bubbling water. Bubble for a couple of moments, at that point strain into a little dish and keep warm. Serve the hamburger in thick cuts, with sauce as an afterthought.
6. Formula TIPS
7. COOK MEAT PERFECTLY
8. For more extraordinary meat, focus on an inner temperature of 55C while slow cooking. For all around done, focus on 75C.

# 14. Slow-roasted courgettes with fennel & orzo

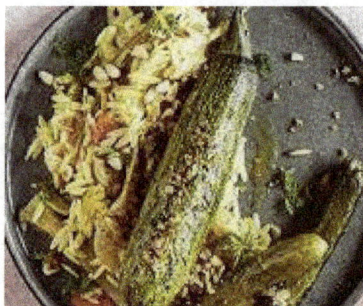

Prep: 25 mins | Cook: 2 hrs. and 10 mins | Easy | Serves 2

## *Ingredients*

- touch of saffron
- 1/2 bulb of fennel , cut
- 100g cherry tomatoes , split
- 1 straight leaf
- 2 tbsp. olive oil
- spot of dried stew drops
- 120ml dry white wine
- 4-6 child to medium-sized courgettes
- 1 lemon , zested
- 50g sourdough breadcrumbs
- 200g orzo
- 1 tbsp. pine nuts , toasted
- 1 tbsp. ricotta
- modest bunch of dill

## Technique

1. Put the saffron in a little bowl and cover with 1/2 tbsp. of bubbling water. Heat oven to 180C/160C fan/gas 4. Put the fennel in a broiling tin with the tomatoes and sound leaf, shower over some oil, season and throw along with the bean stew drops. Pour over the wine. Prick the courgettes done with a fork and spot on top of the fennel. Sprinkle with somewhat more oil, at that point season and cover with foil.
2. Cook for 1/2 - 2 hrs., turning the courgettes partially through, eliminating the foil for the last 5 mins. The courgettes ought to be delicate. Lift the courgettes from the container and put away.
3. In the mean time, heat 1 tbsp. olive oil in a skillet over a medium heat. Add a large portion of the lemon zing and breadcrumbs, and tenderly fry until the bread is brilliant and crunchy. Put away.
4. Cook the orzo in a skillet of bubbling water until still somewhat firm, at that point channel. Throw with the fennel, tomatoes, pine nuts, the saffron and its water. Season.
5. Split the orzo among plates and add a large portion of the ricotta to each, shower with olive oil and sprinkle with ocean salt. Top with the courgettes and disperse over the breadcrumbs, remaining lemon zing and branches of dill.
6. Works out in a good way For
7. Tomato, burrata and expansive bean salad
8. Squashed cannellini beans with shriveled greens and seared artichokes

9. Singed nectarine and prosciutto panzanella.

# 15. Bourbon & honey-glazed brisket with soured cream & chive mash

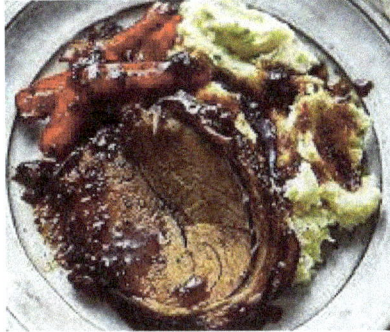

Prep: 15 mins | Cook: 8 hrs. | More effort | Serves 6-8

## Ingredients

- 3 tbsp. vegetable oil
- 2-2½ kg piece meat brisket , rolled and tied (request that your butcher do this for you)
- 1 tbsp. smoked paprika
- 1 tbsp. English mustard powder
- 2 tsp. dried onion powder
- 1 tsp. ground cinnamon
- squeeze dried ground cloves
- 6 tbsp. light brown delicate sugar
- 100g nectar
- 50ml whiskey bourbon, in addition to 2 tbsp.
- 2 red onions , cut
- 4 sound leaves

- 4-6 little carrots , stripped and split or quartered lengthways or 300g Chantenay carrots
- 100ml red wine vinegar
- For the soured cream and chive pound
- 4-6 large preparing potatoes , unpeeled
- 250g soured cream
- 75g spread , in addition to extra to serve
- sprinkle of milk
- little pack chives , chopped

### Strategy

1. Heat 1 tbsp. oil in a large, profound flameproof broiling tin or in your largest flameproof meal dish. Season the meat well and burn in the tin until pleasantly browned all finished, adding the leftover oil to the dish if necessary. Then, blend the paprika, mustard powder, onion powder, cinnamon, cloves, 2 tbsp. sugar, 2 tbsp. nectar and 2 tbsp. of the bourbon in a little bowl with a liberal measure of salt and pepper. Lift out the hamburger and disperse the onions and inlet leaves over the base of the dish, pour in 100ml water and set the meat back on top. Brush the flavor paste everywhere on the meat. Will keep chilled for as long as a day.
2. Heat oven to 150C/130C fan/gas 2. Wrap the tin firmly in a couple of sheets of foil, or cover with a top, and heat for 6-7 hrs., turning more than once during cooking, spooning the juices over the meat and garnish up with a sprinkle more water if the lower part of the dish is dry.

3. Increment the temperature to 200C/180C fan/gas 6. Throw the carrots with the onions around the meat, season at that point cover again with the foil. Penetrate the potatoes a couple of times each and place on the rack underneath the hamburger. Cook for a further 45 mins.

4. Then, pour the leftover sugar, bourbon, nectar and vinegar into a container. In the event that there is bunches of fluid in the tin, add the majority of this as well (yet leave some so the meat doesn't dry out). Season and air pocket to make a tacky coating. Uncover the meat and carrots, brush with the bourbon coating and cook for another 15 mins until the meat is dull, lustrous and delicate, and the carrots and potatoes are delicate. Eliminate from the oven, cover the meat freely with foil and leave to rest for 15 mins.

5. Put the potatoes in a bowl and, when sufficiently cool to deal with, use kitchen scissors to cut them into pieces – you need to save the skin in the pound for additional flavor however any large pieces will be chewy so attempt to separate it however much as could reasonably be expected with the scissors, at that point squash well with a potato masher. Add the soured cream, margarine, milk and the vast majority of the chives, season truly well and crush once more. Move to a bowl and top with a handle of spread and the excess chives. To serve, either cut into thick, delicate cuts or shred the meat with two forks, disposing of any string as you go. Present with

the crush, carrots and onions and spoon over the juices.
6. Works out positively For
7. Thai green curry cook chicken
8. Stuffed butternut squash
9. Darkened dish salmon with avocado and mango salsa.

# 16. Sweet corn fritters with slow-cooked tomatoes

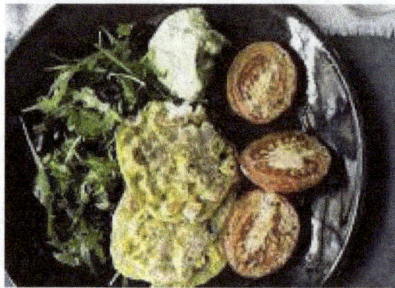

Prep: 30 mins | Cook: 40 mins | Easy | Serves 4

## Ingredients
- 6 large, ready plum tomatoes , divided
- spot of sugar
- avocado cream, (see lower part of pag) to serve
- For the wastes

- 450g sweet corn - utilize new, frozen (thawed out) or canned (depleted)
- 175g plain flour
- 1 tsp. heating powder
- 2 eggs and 2 yolks, beaten
- 125ml milk
- 25g margarine , softened
- 2 spring onions , finely chopped
- ½ red bean stew , deseeded and finely diced
- juice ½ lime
- 25g feta cheddar , disintegrated
- 1 tbsp. each chopped basil and parsley
- olive oil , for fricasseeing
- For the olive serving of mixed greens
- 200g large dark olives , stoned and chopped
- 4 large modest bunches rocket
- sprinkle olive oil
- crush lime juice

## Technique

1. Heat oven to 150C/130C fan/gas 2. Season the tomatoes; add a spot of sugar and meal for around 40 mins. This will focus all their regular pleasantness and flavor.
2. In the case of using new corn, strip away the husks, cut the parts off with a blade, and at that point cook in bubbling water for 4-5 mins. Channel. Filter the flour and preparing powder into a bowl, making a well in the middle. Add the eggs, yolks and a large portion of the milk. Beat until smooth; at that point slowly rush in the excess milk and margarine. Crease in the corn, spring onions, bean stew, lime juice, feta

and spices. Season, remembering the feta is somewhat pungent.

3. Heat and delicately oil a weighty based skillet. Drop 2-3 loaded tbsp. of the combination into the container and fry over a medium heat for around 3 mins each side, or until brilliant brown and cooked through. Move to the oven and rehash with the leftover player – makes around 16. They will save well like this for a couple of hours, in the event that you need to make them ahead.

4. For the plate of mixed greens, blend the olives, spices and rocket together. Shower with oil and lime juice. Serve the wastes with the plate of mixed greens, tomato parts and avocado cream.

5. Formula TIPS

6. AVOCADO CREAM

7. Put 2 medium stripped and generally chopped avocados, juice 1 large lime, ½ little garlic clove squashed and ½ tbsp. olive oil in a food processor. Whizz to a smooth purée and overlap in 2 tbsp. crème fraîche. Taste and season, adding more lime juice in the event that you figure the flavor could be somewhat more honed.

# 17.  Venetian duck ragu

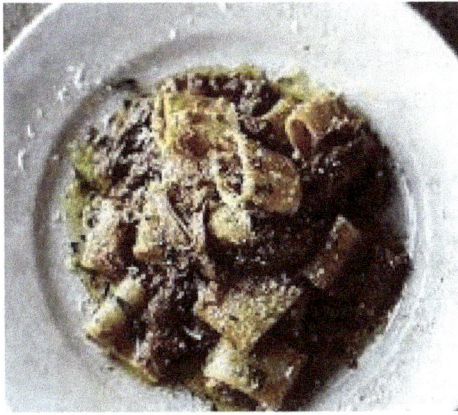

Prep: 15 mins| Cook: 2 hrs. and 30 mins | Easy |
Serves 6

## *Ingredients*

- 1 tbsp. olive oil
- 4 duck legs
- 2 onions, finely chopped
- 2 fat garlic cloves, squashed
- 2 tsp. ground cinnamon
- 2 tsp. plain flour
- 250ml red wine
- 2 x 400g jars chopped tomatoes
- 1 chicken stock solid shape, made up to 250ml
- 3 rosemary branches, leaves picked and chopped
- 2 straight leaves
- 1 tsp. sugar
- 2 tbsp. milk
- 600g paccheri or pappardelle pasta
- parmesan, ground, to serve

## Strategy

1. Heat the oil in a large container. Add the duck legs and brown on all sides for around 10 mins. Eliminate to a plate and put away. Add the onions to the container and cook for 5 mins until relaxed. Add the garlic and cook for a further 1 min, at that point mix in the cinnamon and flour and cook for a further min. Return the duck to the dish, add the wine, tomatoes, stock, spices, sugar and preparing. Bring to a stew, at that point bring down the heat, cover with a top and cook for 2 hrs., blending from time to time.

2. Cautiously lift the duck legs out of the sauce and spot on a plate – they will be delicate so do whatever it takes not to lose any of the meat. Pull off and dispose of the fat, at that point shred the meat with 2 forks and dispose of the bones. Add the meat back to the sauce with the milk and stew, revealed, for a further 10-15 mins while you cook the pasta.

3. Cook the pasta adhering to pack guidelines, at that point channel, holding some the pasta water, and add the pasta to the ragu. Mix to cover all the pasta in the sauce and cook for 1 min more, adding a sprinkle of cooking fluid on the off chance that it looks dry. Present with ground Parmesan, in the event that you like.

4. Works out positively For

5. Panna cotta with apricot compote

6. Tart fennel and rocket salad

# 18. Low 'n' slow rib steak with Cuban mojo salsa

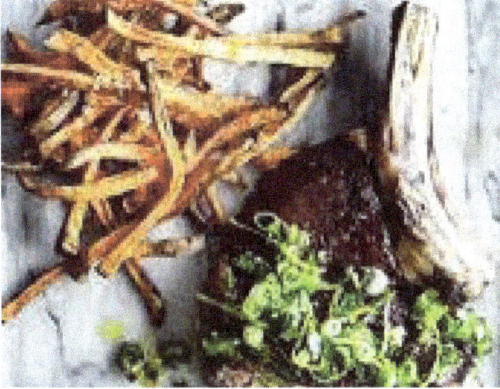

Preparation and cooking time | Prep: 20 mins | Cook: 3 hrs. and 20 mins | More effort | Serves 2

## Ingredients

- 1 rib steak on the bone or côte du boeuf (about 800g)
- 1 tbsp. rapeseed oil
- 1 garlic clove
- 2 thyme branches
- 25g margarine , chopped into little pieces
- yam fries
- a dressed plate of mixed greens , to serve
- For the magic salsa
- 2 limes
- 1 little orange
- ½ little bundle mint , finely chopped
- little bundle coriander , finely chopped
- 4 spring onions , finely chopped
- 1 little garlic clove , squashed

- 1 fat green bean stew , finely chopped
- 4 tbsp. additional virgin rapeseed oil or olive oil

## Technique

1. Leave the hamburger at room temperature for around 1 hr. before you cook it. Heat oven to 60C/40C fan/gas 1/4 on the off chance that you like your meat medium uncommon, or 65C/45C fan/gas 1/4 for medium. (Cooking at these low temperatures will be more precise in an electric oven than in a gas one. In the case of using gas, put the oven on the most reduced setting you have, and know that the cooking time might be more limited.)

2. Put the unseasoned hamburger in a weighty based ovenproof skillet. Cook in the oven for 3 hrs. undisturbed.

3. Then, make the salsa. Zing the limes and orange into a bowl. Slice each down the middle and spot, cut-side down, in a hot skillet. Cook for a couple of mins until the organic products are burned, at that point crushes the juice into the bowl. Add different ingredients and season well.

4. At the point when the hamburger is cooked, it should look dry on a superficial level, and dull pink in shading. On the off chance that you have a meat thermometer, test the inside temperature – it ought to be 58-60C. Eliminate the dish from the oven and set over a high heat on the hob. Add the oil and singe the meat on the two sides for a couple of mins until caramelized. Singe the fat for a couple of mins as well. Crush the garlic clove with the

impact point of your hand and add this to the container with the thyme and spread. At the point when the spread is frothing, spoon it over the meat and cook for another 1-2 mins. Move the meat to a warm plate, cover with foil, and leave to rest for 5-10 mins. Cut away from the bone and into cuts prior to presenting with the salsa, fries and salad.

5. Works out positively For
6. Chimichurri sauce
7. Heated thin fries
8. Yam fries

# 19. Slow-roast pork rolls with apple chili chutney

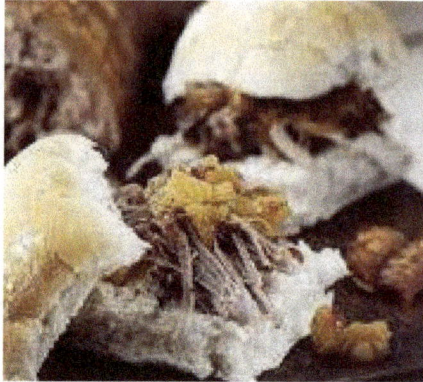

Prep: 15 mins | Cook: 6 hrs. | Easy| Serves 6 - 8

## *Ingredients*
- 2.5kg/5lb 8oz pork shoulder joint, scored and tied (we utilized a tied carvery joint from Waitrose, bone in one end and rolled and tied at opposite end)
- 2 tsp. thyme leaves
- 1 tsp. fennel seed
- 1 tbsp. olive oil
- buttered delicate bread moves , to serve
- For the apple stew chutney
- 1 tbsp. olive oil
- 2 onions , finely chopped
- 1-2 red chilies , deseeded and finely chopped
- 4 eating apples , stripped, cored and cut into little pieces
- 4 tbsp. juice vinegar
- 4 tbsp. caster sugar

- 1 thyme twig, leaves picked

## *Strategy*

1. Heat oven to 240C/220C fan/gas 9. Sit the pork in a large cooking tin. In the event that the skin isn't as of now scored for you, score it with a little, sharp blade. Combine as one the thyme, fennel seeds, oil and 1 tsp. salt with a decent crushing of dark pepper. Rub this ludicrous and finishes of the pork. Broil for 30 mins, at that point cover the entire tin with a large sheet of foil, diminish the oven temperature to 140C/120C fan/gas 1 and return the pork to the oven for a further 5 hrs.

2. While the pork is cooking, make the chutney. Heat the oil in a large pot. Relax the onion and bean stew together for 10-15 mins. When delicate, mix in the apple lumps, vinegar and sugar with 50ml water. Cover and cook over a low heat for 15-20 mins, blending sporadically, until the apple is exceptionally delicate. Rush a large portion of the apple combination with a hand blender, or scoop half into a food processor and whizz until smooth, prior to mixing once more into the container with the leaves from the thyme twig.

3. Take the pork from the oven – the meat ought to be delicate – and increment the temperature to 240C/220C fan/gas 9. At the point when the oven has arrived at temperature, dispose of the foil and set the pork back in for 30 mins to fresh up the skin a bit. For truly fresh popping, eliminate the skin from the meat, envelop the meat by foil to keep warm, and return just the

skin to the oven for 30 mins. A few forks to shred the pork from the joint. Sandwich in delicate buttered moves with apple bean stew chutney, warm or at room temperature. Present with bits of fresh snapping as an afterthought.

# 20. Beef bourguignon with celeriac mash

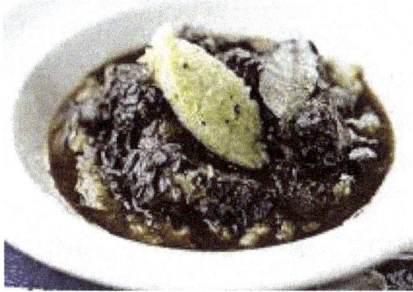

Prep: 20 mins |Cook:3 hrs. and 15 mins | Easy |
Serves 4

## Ingredients

- 1 tbsp. goose fat
- 600g shin meat, cut into large lumps
- 100g smoked dirty bacon, cut
- 350g shallot or pearl onions, stripped
- 250g chestnut mushrooms (around 20)
- 2 garlic cloves, cut
- 1 bouquet garni (see ability beneath)
- 1 tbsp. tomato purée
- 750ml jug red wine, Burgundy is acceptable
- For the celeriac pound
- 600g (around 1) celeriac
- 2 tbsp. olive oil, in addition to a glug
- 1 or 2 rosemary and thyme twigs
- 2 cove leaves
- 4 cardamom units

## Strategy

1. Heat a large goulash dish and add 1 tbsp. goose fat.

2. Season 600g large lumps of shin hamburger and fry until brilliant brown, around 3-5 mins, at that point turn over and fry the opposite side until the meat is browned all finished, adding more fat if important. Do this in 2-3 clusters, moving the meat to a colander set over a bowl when browned.
3. In a similar skillet, fry 100g cut smoked smudgy bacon, 350g stripped shallots or pearl onions, 250g chestnut mushrooms, 2 cut garlic cloves and 1 bouquet garni until softly browned.
4. Blend in 1 tbsp. tomato purée and cook for a couple of mins, mixing the combination. This enhances the bourguignon and makes an incredible base for the stew. At that point return the meat and any depleted juices to the skillet and mix through.
5. Pour over 750ml container red wine and about 100ml water so the meat bounces up from the fluid, however isn't totally covered. Bring to the bubble and utilize a spoon to scratch the caramelized cooking juices from the lower part of the container – this will give the stew more flavors.
6. Heat oven to 150C/fan 130C/gas 2. Make a cartouche: detach a square of foil somewhat larger than the goulash, organize it in the skillet so it covers the highest point of the stew and trim away any abundance foil. Cook for 3 hrs.
7. On the off chance that the sauce looks watery, eliminate the meat and veg with an opened spoon, and put away. Cook the sauce over a

high heat for a couple of mins until the sauce has thickened a little, at that point returns the hamburger and vegetables to the dish.

8. To make the celeriac squash, strip 600g celeriac and cut into blocks. Heat 2 tbsp. olive oil in a large griddle. Tip in the celeriac and fry for 5 mins until it becomes brilliant. Season well with salt and pepper.

9. Mix in 1 or 2 branches of rosemary and thyme, 2 cove leaves and 4 cardamom cases, at that point pour over 200ml water, enough to almost cover the celeriac. Turn the heat to low, in part cover the container and leave to stew for 25-30 mins.

10.    After 25-30 mins, the celeriac ought to be delicate and the majority of the water will have vanished. Channel away any excess water, at that point eliminate the spice branches, sound and cardamom units.

11.    Daintily smash with a potato masher, at that point get done with a glug of olive oil and season to taste.

12.    Spoon the hamburger bourguignon into serving bowls and spot a large spoonful of the celeriac pound on top. Enhancement with one of the narrows leaves, on the off chance that you like.

13.    Formula TIPS

14.    MAKE AHEAD

15.    Attempt to make this dish a day ahead of time, at that point slowly reheat in the oven. You'll see that the flavors will truly grow for the time being and the dish will be more extravagant and more develop.

16.     Skill - BOUQUET GARNI
17.     To make a bouquet garni, utilize a piece of string to two or three rosemary, thyme and parsley twigs and a small bunch of inlet leaves. Eliminate from the dish toward the finish of cooking and dispose of.
18.     Hamburger SHIN
19.     Hamburger shin is an incredible cut for slow-cooking. It's acceptable worth and the waves of fat going through it guarantee that it doesn't dry out. You could likewise utilize wild hog, which gives a truly unique flavor.
20.     TIP - PEELING ONIONS
21.     To strip shallots or pearl onions rapidly, place in an astonish and pour bubbling water. Leave for a couple of moments, at that point channel and the skins will sneak off.
22.     Works out positively For:
23.     Irish soft drink bread

# 21. Slow cooked Ossobuco

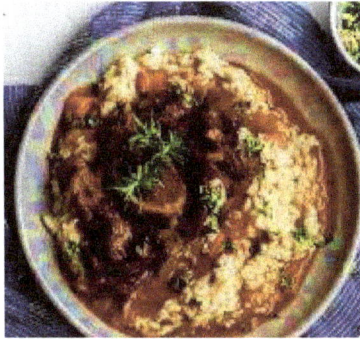

Prep tim2: 3 hours | Serves 2

## Ingredients

- veal or meat shin 8 pieces around 4-5cm thick, cut across the bone (request that the butcher do this)
- plain flour 100g, all around prepared
- olive oil
- onions 2 enormous, finely chopped
- carrots 4, stripped and finely chopped
- celery 4 sticks, managed and finely chopped
- garlic 4 cloves, squashed
- white wine 300ml
- sound leaves 3
- thyme 3 twigs
- veal or chicken stock 1.5-2 liters
- GERMOLATA
- lemon 1, zested
- garlic 1 cloves, finely chopped
- level leaf parsley a little bundle, finely chopped

**DIRECTION:**

1. Heat the oven to 180C/fan 160C/gas 4. Season the veal pieces well, at that point delicately dust in the prepared flour.


2. Heat 2 tbsp. oil in a non-stick dish on a high heat, and fry the meat in groups for a couple of moments on each side until brilliant earthy colored. Move to a plate and rehash with the excess pieces. Add another tbsp. oil to the dish, on the off chance that you need to, while singing.

3. Lower the heat to medium and add tbsp. oil to the container in the event that you need to, add the onion, carrot, celery and a touch of salt. Fry for 10 minutes until exceptionally delicate and clear.

4. Add the garlic and fry for one more moment prior to pouring in the wine. Stew until decreased considerably, scraping up any pieces from the lower part of the skillet. Add the narrows leaves and thyme.

5. Move the meat, the veg and the fluid from the griddle to a huge goulash with a cover. Add the stock to simply cover the meat, season well and bring to a stew.

6. Cover with the top and move to the oven. Cook for 2 hours until the meat is truly delicate (you may require longer for hamburger shin).

7. Combine the gremolata ingredients as one with a touch of salt and dissipate over the ossobuco. Present with crush, polenta, or saffron risotto.

8. Instructions to store it: serve straight away, or leave to cool to room temperature and move to Tupperware boxes, and freeze. It will save for a half year. Defrost in the cooler expedite and reheat.

# Conclusion

Thank you for going through recipes in this book.
Slow cooker is easy to use and it just needs practice.
Try the incredible recipes in this book and enjoy.
I wish you good luck!

CPSIA information can be obtained
at www.ICGtesting.com
Printed in the USA
LVHW060904030621
688874LV00047B/150

9 781802 005172